Vital Sensation Manual

UNIT THREE:
KINGDOMS

Based on
The Sensation Method
& Classical Homeopathy

Written
by
Melissa Burch, CCH

Edited by Ingrid Dankmeyer, Didi Pershouse and Sharon Willis

Cover Design by Chetana Deorah

Text Design by Janet Innes and George Papargyris

Published by
Inner Health, Inc.
175 Harvey St., #13
Cambridge, MA 02140
(617) 491-3374
melissa@innerhealth.us
www.innerhealth.us

TABLE OF CONTENTS

A. DOCTRINE OF SIGNATURES

> *Any sensation or phenomenon arising during a proving is but a seed that has always existed within us, a seed that has never before germinated and flowered. Just as the sun and rain nurture the seedling so the proving fosters an embryonic side of our nature. Thus we gain insight into a previously hidden aspect of ourselves. Simultaneously we may also perceive an aspect of the natural universe previously hidden from us. Thus if we prove Scorpion we experience the inner perspective of a scorpion. If we prove Silica we experience the inner nature of a rock or a grain of sand.*
>
> Jeremy Sherr
> "The Dynamics and Methodology of Homoeopathic Provings"

The Doctrine of Signatures is a controversial idea in homeopathy. Hahnemann warned against it in its simplest form. The idea that Orchis root, a substance shaped like a testicle will restore manly vigor is simplistic and superficial. Vithoulkas also lamented that to prescribe zebra to a patient who only wants to wear striped shirts is absurd. However, understanding a remedy and its connection to the substance and studying its qualities, attributes and environment in nature can be very useful. It is also necessary to understand why a patient does something and how that connects to the prescription. In essence everything is interconnected. Through homeopathy the practitioner tries to understand the state of the patient and the effects of the remedy in its totality, which means acknowledging that there is a connection between the substance and nature, and how that relates to the patient in an individualistic expression.

Boger in "The Study of Materia Medica" writes:

> "According to the Doctrine of Signatures they have a meaning for us if we are only wise enough to see and use them. When we bear in mind that the universe moves forward in obedience to laws which work harmoniously and that every part thereof bears a definite relation to every other part, no fact however insignificant remains without value."

The Doctrine of Signature can be a way to understand the different kingdoms. What are the similar characteristics of all animals, of all plants and of all minerals as they are understood in nature? In addition, after extensive study of the Materia Medica, common symptoms were recognized from remedies of the same kingdom. There is a collective state or pattern of behavior based on a specific kingdom. Patients will express general characteristics of the plant, animal or mineral kingdom.

In provings, individual states are produced by remedies, which are connected to the source of the remedy and represent the spirit of that substance. For example, Lachesis has left sidedness which can be related to the fact that this snake has all its organs on the left side of the body. J.H. Clarke in "Dictionary of Practical Materia Medica" writes: "As the fox is probably the longest-winded of all animals, the Doctrine of Signatures pointed to his lungs as a likely remedy for shortness of breath."

The qualities of plants, animals or minerals are part of the expression of the individual state or what needs to be cured in the patient. The homeopath needs to listen for this information and recognize the language of an animal or plant or mineral expressed by a human being so that the selection of the remedy can be narrowed to a specific kingdom. This understanding of homeopathy and the language of kingdoms opened homeopathy to the natural world beyond its Materia Medica, provings, repertories and symptom-based analysis.

In the past a homeopath could be looking at Lac caninum, Argentum metallicum and Staphysagria for one prescription, and this is where there is a lot of confusion in homeopathy. In the effort to understand kingdoms some of this differentiating will become easier.

B. CLASSIFICATION OF THE KINGDOMS

The significance of this method is that homeopathy becomes a classification system instead of just being based on a collection of symptoms. Traditionally homeopaths have selected remedies according to symptoms and have had to differentiate from several different remedies which could come from any of the kingdoms.

This method uses a classification process in order to find the patient's remedy. The homeopath now asks: What kingdom does the patient express? Is it the plant, animal or mineral kingdom? This has expanded the use of many smaller or unknown remedies with much more accuracy and effectiveness.

The approach requires knowing that the Level of Sensation in the casetaking is where the patient will speak in more specific non-human terms so that the kingdom, the sub-kingdom and the source of their remedy will be confirmed. Throughout the case the patient may use language from all the kingdoms, so it is important to be sure that the Vital Sensation or symptom that connects the mind and body is confirmed and explored at the Level of Sensation in order to find the specific kingdom. A case that focuses mainly on a human situation like marital infidelity will not be able to confirm the specific kingdom. The Vital Sensation, which is non-human specific, will give the clues necessary to find the accurate kingdom.

C. THE DIFFERENT QUALITIES OF THE KINGDOMS

Each kingdom has its own distinctive nature. Patients who need plant remedies will have great sensitivity and reactivity. Patients who need mineral remedies will have issues with structure. Patients who need animal remedies will focus on competition and struggle for survival. In addition to the plant, mineral and animal kingdoms there are nosodes, sarcodes and imponderables to consider.

A patient may come with the chief complaint of heartburn. The person who needs a plant remedy will say it is burning pain like a tearing apart and scattered sensation. When the homeopath inquires about the opposite sensation they will say it feels like everything is bound together (Leguminosae family). A patient who needs a mineral remedy may talk about how the burning sensation of the heartburn feels like a pressure which comes when they are overworked and they feel pressured when the boss gives them a deadline they can't meet. A patient who needs an animal remedy will talk about the heartburn as if someone took a burning knife and stabbed them. They constantly feel they are being attacked by their boss and are sure that to succeed they have to be the very best.

Minerals

Minerals at their deepest core experience emptiness. The sensation is that the structure is lacking or forming. The mineral experience is either to have or to lose.

The Period

•

Newtonian thinking:
The smallest particle
The sensation is does it exist or not exist
Existential question

Is the sensation about existence?
What does it mean to exist?
How to exist?
In relationship, identity, work, etc.

Plants

The sensation itself is expressed as a life experience and as a reaction to the patients' experiences. The feeling is a sensation and it is experienced directly in their chief complaint, relationships, dreams, emotions, work, etc. The sensation is happening within, the phenomenon happens within. The sensation exists mostly within a relationship of its opposite.

The Line

Sacred Geometry
The line goes out and must come back to itself.
Sensation is itself and its opposite.
Does the sensation come back to itself (through its opposite)?

Animals

Something is happening from the outside. For example, you are killing me, pursuing me, dominating me. They will give sensations but no opposite. There will be a fight with the sensation. For example: the sensation is pressure but no opposite (only loose/relax with no energy). The pressure is killing me. I have to fight with the pressure. It is me vs. the other, strong vs. weak, etc.

The Spiral

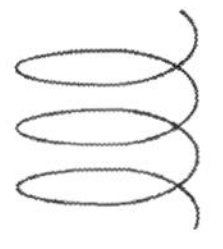

Quantum Physics

What happens in one place at one time affects everything.
A single creature communicates to the whole species.
The whole species communicates to the single creature.
For example: One monkey learns to wash a potato on one island, all the monkeys on the island learn to wash their potatoes, then all monkeys can wash potatoes.

Collective Consciousness

Is this why often times the name of the animal can be told or explained clearly to the homeopath?

The consciousness of the species is able to be identified and expressed directly by the patient. The sensation of the animal or a specific species can be expressed because of their relationships to each other and to the human race.

The themes of aggression, competition, survival, and so forth can be expressed through the sensations because of the collective consciousness. Something coming from the outside is the beginning of separation or individual, which perhaps began as a consciousness in animals. An animal can carry its relationships to other animals in its consciousness (its prey, its aggressor and other animal characteristics). It is important not to confuse an animal mentioned by the patient with the remedy required. It could be an animal in relationship to or similar to the one described or mentioned.

NOSODES

The Pyramid

The nosode is a collective consciousness expressed in the miasm.

Disease is a human/animal/plant drama (which may come from bacteria, parasite, virus, organ/cellular/mind imbalance, etc.), but cannot be isolated from time and space or from its interaction with an organism. The miasm is a specific drama (or disease) with a collective identity. Is the miasm theme or drama expressed throughout all the sensations?

The difference of kingdoms at a superficial level is very confusing. For example, the issue for the patient could be focused on relationships, which is a more human specific problem. A plant may express the hurt as a structure breaking apart, but the homeopath needs to examine if the emphasis is on breaking and coming apart as a sensation that is characteristic and repeated as a Vital Sensation on the mind and body. It is not about the structure itself but about a sensation felt within the patient throughout areas of his life. Then a plant remedy is required. It is a specific and repeated sensitivity and reaction. It is not a representation of a feeling but a direct sensation felt by the patient, which will be expressed in more non-human specific language. In a mineral, the relationship problem may be expressed as a hurt or sensitivity which will not be a specific sensation but more about the language of structure and the patient's role in the relationship. In animals it will be me versus someone else, such as "I am worthless or he is worthless." There will be an issue of victim and aggressor, which are both sides of the same coin.

Where does the problem of the case exist?

Problem area	Kingdom
Structure	Mineral
Survival	Animal
Sensitivity	Plant

D. PLANT KINGDOM

The basic quality of a plant is sensitivity. It is a living organism rooted to the soil, unable to move, and essentially can only face and react to physical challenges like the weather. The plant needs to be sensitive to changes in the external environment and also capable of adapting to these changes in order to survive. These features of being sensitive, affected by many things, and adjusting and adapting to these things are qualities of plant remedies.

Choice of clothing – preferring flowery and irregular patterns – may reflect this sensitivity. Handwriting may be rounded and disorganized reflecting more of an "irregular pattern." Manner of speech may be disorganized: talking about other people's complaints, describing their problems incompletely, and in no particular order. In the follow-ups it might begin abruptly. This type may be very descriptive in expressing how intensely they feel most things. The complaints often have a rapid onset and changing nature, with many modalities. The causative factor is often emotional or physical, a particular strain or hurt. These observations are only clues, and it is important not to make a distinction until the Level of Sensation is reached where more non-human language is expressed and the plant kingdom can be confirmed more directly.

The expressions they use are: "I am affected by or sensitive to…" "This hurts me," "I can't bear this," "This touches me." These expressions show their focus on their sensitivity, softness and emotions. Feelings and the fear of being hurt are most important to them. They are easily affected and can have abrupt mood changes. Their dreams can be varied (of plants, greenery, nature, music, art, etc.) and more influenced by the day's occurrences because of their sensitivity. The Plant Kingdom experiences death as extreme suffering and pain.

A specific sensation or reaction will be expressed in all aspects of the patient's life (interests, stressful situations, relationships, etc.) and most of the time will be accompanied by the same gestures. Remedies from a particular plant family will share at least one common sensation or type of pain. The Vital Sensation of a particular plant family can be expressed in four different ways: the sensation itself, its passive reaction, its active reaction, and its compensation. For example if the sensation is that of being injured or hurt (the Compositae family), the passive reaction is to feel dazed (Arnica), the active reaction is to strike back (Chamomilla) and the compensation is to become tough enough to take any hurt (Arnica). All remedies of a particular family will have all these reactions but some remedies are better known for a particular reaction.

The common theme in plants is sensitivity and reactivity, and it is not a mental state but a general expression of a deeper vital disturbance. For example, in the Loganiaceae family, which has the remedies Nux vomica, Gelsemium and Ignatia, it is not obvious what is common to these remedies. Nux vomica is bossy, fastidious, impatient and irritable. Gelsemium is nervous, tremulous, drowsy, and cannot take bad news. Ignatia has grief, disappointment or shock and has to hold everything within. The common sensation in all these remedies is shock, and the difference is how each remedy perceives and experiences this sensation. Each remedy is differentiated by its miasm, which has its own pace, depth and degree of desperation and reaction, which again can be confirmed at the Level of Sensation.

In Nux Vomica there is a feeling of "how can I recover from this shock?" (the Vital Sensation). The situation is critical and the individual has to come out of it as quickly as he can, otherwise he is sunk. For example: The stock market has fallen and I must recover quickly and reach a position of comfort. Then I am fine. This indicates the Typhoid miasm.

In Gelsemium the feeling that "I cannot withstand the shock, and I am too weak and must avoid anything that causes the shock." He avoids shock. He goes to the toilet and shuts the door, trembles and goes to sleep. Tell him that he must give a speech and he avoids it. This indicates the Sycotic miasm.

Ignatia perceives that she cannot avoid the shock. A woman with three small children wakes and finds her husband dead! There is no way she can avoid it. It is complete chaos. Her whole life has gone from total order to total chaos. She perceives the shock as chaos. In a situation of shock she has to be in control. This indicates the Cancer miasm.

The common sensation is shock, and each remedy has its own pace, depth and degree of desperation and reaction. Though it shares the common sensation of the family, it experiences this sensation in a different way, a Typhoid way, a Sycotic way and a Cancer way. The way the patient perceives their chief complaint and Vital Sensation will identify the miasm and help to select the specific remedy from a particular plant family.

In order to find the specific remedy from a plant family, it is important to find the Vital Sensation – whether it is reactive, passive, compensated or a more general expression – and then to perceive the miasm or the depth and intensity of how the patient copes in the different areas of his life. It is important to understand the patient's Vital Sensation at the Level of Sensation, where it is not about emotional problems but about their sensitivity and reaction. For example, Bellis perennis has issues with trauma (Compositae family) which it must face and keep under control (Cancer miasm). When the prescription is based on the Vital Sensations it is more likely to be accurate.

The study of the sensations of each plant family is an ongoing process. Dr. Sankaran has charted numerous families which are available in *Insights into Plants Vol. 1 and 2* as well as his latest schema, *Sankaran's Schema [2005 Edition],* and in the computer program, *Vital Quest.* Other homeopaths are also researching the common sensations in the different plant families, and much of this information is being clinically evaluated and shared in the homeopathic community.

In some plant families there are only a few known remedies, so that it was not possible to have a remedy designated for every miasm. There are some plant families where using the super order revealed a common theme, which turned out to share a similar sensation throughout the family.

Note: There are some plants that will have animal characteristics, such as the Nephenthes family which has Drosera, with the feeling of being attacked, suffocated, etc.

E. ANIMAL KINGDOM

The main themes of the animal remedies are:

- Issues of survival or threat to their life. They will kill me, cut me, bite me, rip me off, tear me apart, pounce on me, desire to hide, etc. The fear of death is expressed as a fear of being attacked, a violent death, killed, murdered, chased.

- Victim and aggressor. They feel victimized by people or the illness. People are doing this to me. The illness is doing this to me. The illness is attacking me. They use words like teased, bullied, victimized, harassed, nagged, abused, forced, torture, fighting, etc. There are themes of strong and weak, predator and prey, one versus the other, me against you, persecutor and persecuted.

- Hierarchy. Who is superior or inferior? They are dominating me, overpowering me, above me, dictating to me. I'm under someone, low level, etc.

- Animal references. I feel caged, trapped, bound, captured, chained, shackled, imprisoned, want to be free, escape, etc.

- Sexuality and Attractiveness. There is a need to attract attention in their behavior and appearance. They can be very attractive and seductive. They can also feel dirty about themselves. They want to be the center of attention, can be loquacious and communicative. Attraction and sexuality are very important for the propagation of the species.

- Competition. This struggle is core to survival in the animal world.

- Split within one self. Contradiction of will. This conflict is about the two different sides of themselves: the animal side and the human side. Many times the human side seems to have contempt for the animal within. The split exists within the self: "I hate myself," "Me versus myself," "I am disgusted with myself." They may express it as: "human beings do...," "Human beings are so cruel," "I feel split up," "I jump at them," "I am not good enough," etc.

- Jealousy.

- Need to belong to a group.

- Lack of morality. They can be deceitful or malicious.

There is a connection with the source. There is a fear, fascination or aversion to animals or to one in particular. It may appear only in dreams. In most of the cases the patient will give a good hint by showing an intense connection with the source animal.

The homeopath should be very careful about when to ask leading questions related to the source animal. If it is asked prematurely, it may not lead to the specific sub-kingdom and source for the patient or it may be to an animal that is not the remedy required. Only after exploring all the aspects of the case (like fears, dreams, interests and hobbies, intense situations, job, relationship, etc.) and the Level of Sensation is confirmed, then the qualities of the source animal will easily connect to the patient.

A simple question like "how do you react to animals?" may unfold the whole connection. For example, most of the cases of reptiles will show intense fear or dreams or liking for snakes. Or the patient belonging to the bird sub-kingdom would show intense liking or hatred for birds. The next question would be to find out if there is any specific bird that he likes or dislikes. This would lead us further to the specific source.

The patient may mention many animals, but throughout the case the energy of the animal and the energy of the patient should be compared. He may mention other animals just for their specific quality but they do not resonate to it. For example, he mentions a horse for its power, but the patient needs a different animal that has power. The patient may also be describing qualities of the predator animal and they need the prey. For example, they may describe the eagle but need the mouse. The way to confirm is to see if anything does not fit. For example in the patient's description of the eagle he talks about how small and frightened he feels while soaring through the sky.

When there is not a clear cut Vital Sensation or many Vital Sensations, then think of an animal remedy. However, be aware that it could also be a mineral remedy but the themes of structure will have to be in the case. The Vital Sensation leads to the issue of survival, victim-aggressor, hierarchy, competition, attractiveness, etc. Every aspect of the patient's life can be narrowed down to these issues.

Among the animal remedies, different sub-kingdoms, e.g. snakes, insects, birds, etc. will each represent its own characteristic features. Some points that help us in the process of differentiation are:

- Connection with the source and relation with other animals
- The kind of attack feeling
- Group feeling, belonging to a herd
- Fast pace, hyperactivity
- Miasm
- Sexuality
- Other qualities, for example there are solitary birds and mammals which express more loner themes.

There are some specific animal remedies that have been classified by miasms and can be a very rough guide to choosing the sub-kingdom and remedy.

For example:
Acute miasm: Lyssin
Sycotic or near Sycotic miasms (Malaria or Ringworm): many Mammals
Tubercular miasm: Arachneda and Insecta
Syphilitic or near Syphilitic miasm (Cancer, Leprosy): predator mammals like Lac leoninum, Reptiles

Steps to casetaking if it is an animal remedy:

- From the chief complaint, find the Vital Sensation and then through the different levels (Delusion, Sensation and Energy) find the issues of the animal kingdom repeated over and over.
- Once the animal kingdom is confirmed at the Level of Sensation then the sub-kingdom can be explored.
- Is it more a victim or aggressor feeling (attacking or being attacked)?
- What is the miasm of the case?
- Is there a fast pace like Arachnida (spiders), Insecta (insects) or predator like cheetah?
- Is there a herd mentality like mammals or birds or other species?
- Look for other animal characteristics that will help understand which species is needed.
- Once there is a confirmation of the sub-kingdom, then look for the source. Is there a fear, fascination, aversion or dreams that connect to a specific source? This reference can be a good guiding point to the remedy.
- Always check what doesn't fit. Do not take the animal presented without getting all the qualities and if something doesn't fit then explore this detail thoroughly. In animal cases it is easy to jump to a conclusion when an animal is mentioned by the patient. Be careful.

Note: There are also sea animals which will have many plant characteristics such as the sea anemone, which will be very sensitive and not easily express the animal characteristics.

The animal kingdom is further divided into classes and sub-classes which represent the different types of survival modes.

- Mollusks
- Arachnida
- Insects
- Fishes
- Reptiles
- Birds
- Mammals

Each species has a different survival mode, which can be studied in the repertory, *Materia Medica* and in nature. For example, insects have the following characteristic symptoms when extracted from the repertory: busy, violent, and sudden death (fear of sudden death, delusion he will die suddenly). This is the life of an insect – busy, violent and sudden death. Bees and ants are busy all the time. They inflict violence and get it in return.

Animal Characteristics

Type of attacks:

Cunningness:	Arachnida, Reptiles
Strangulated, constricted, choked:	Reptiles
Attack from behind:	Reptiles

Poisoned:	Reptiles
Open, sky, flying:	Birds
Territory, encroachment	Mammals, Arachnida, Insecta
Shell, protection, cover	Crustacea, Mollusk
Group security	Mammals, Birds
Speed, high pace, hyperactivity, restlessness	Arachnida, Insecta, Amphibian
Power and speed of predator	Mammals, Birds
Clairvoyance	Reptiles
Periodicity	Arachnida
Strong maternal instincts	Mammals, Birds
Breast tenderness before menses	Mammals, Mollusk
Tobacco cravings	Arachnida

F. MINERAL KINGDOM

The central themes common to remedies of the mineral kingdom are structure and organization. The problems arise from a break in structure and organization, breaking of relationships or failure in performance. They tend to be highly organized and very systematic. If the structure is fulfilled then they do not have a problem. The structure has to do with roles and positions, relationships and performance, as well as how much can the patient defend his structure. The lack of structure will be expressed as lack of stamina, support, position, confidence, security, relation, etc. These ideas are human expressions and will be understood in the case at the Level of Delusion.

A mineral remedy should be considered when the Vital Sensation leads to issues of structure and organization, and it is confirmed in every aspect of the patient's life. In addition, if a patient doesn't give you a clear cut Vital Sensation or gives many Vital Sensations, then consider a mineral remedy but also remain open. It could be an animal remedy if there are themes of survival and competition.

The effort now is to understand the mineral kingdom in terms of Source words or non-human specific language. The confusion in minerals is how to differentiate a specific remedy when using situational problems. For example, I feel unsure about who I am. This is very general, and without a deep exploration of what the person means, it could be any number of remedies from Rows one to three of the Periodic Table. The new approach to casetaking where the patient expresses the Level of Sensation and Energy is revealing more specific Source language for the mineral kingdom, which will add to our understanding of the elements.

Common Source words of minerals:

Absorption
Alloy
Analyzing
Backbone
Balance
Base
Basic structure
Bond capacity
Breaking
Brittle
Bulk
Catalyst
Categorizing
Cement
Coins
Collapsing
Compression
Fall
Fire
Fluid
Foundation
Fragile
Fragment
Freezing
Friction
Fusion
Glass
Golden
Gouge
Gravity
Growth
Hard
Heat
Heavy
Predictable
Punctual
Quantifying
Quantity
Radiation
Relatives
Resistance
Rock
Rough
Rusting
Sashes
Schedule
Sliver
Smoke
Smooth
Soft
Solidity

Condense	Height	Sparks
Conduction	Hole	Stable
Construction	Hollow	Standing on your own feet
Corrosion	Impression	Statistics
Crystallization	Iron	Steel
Dead relatives	Lasting	Stone
Dense	Magnetic	Stream
Development	Material	Strength
Disorganized	Metal	Structure
Dissolution	Molecules	Tension
Durable	Nuclear	Unstable
Elastic	Pattern	Vacuum
Electric	Permanent	Vapor
Empty	Pieces	Vibration
Evaporate	Pillar	Weakness

The understanding of stages and rows is to follow many of the ideas of Jan Scholten who organized the mineral kingdom using the Table of Elements. The perception of source language to distinguish the row and stages is being explored by Sankaran and is still in its beginning stages of development.

The Periodic Table is a series of rows and columns. Each row and column has a particular significance. Each column seems to represent a stage of human development and can be examined by understanding the foundation of the structure and the reaction to challenges. Similarly each row has its own understanding.

Up to stage 10 there is a development of these qualities. At stage 10 the structure is complete. As it then progresses further, the structure gradually cannot keep up with that intended function. As it progresses from left to right it becomes more and more rigid and more fixed about the type of structure. Also the remedies get more and more specialized. But along with that they also get more insecure about their structure since they have no choice and they then perceive more and more threat and thus an increasing fear of failure.

ROWS:	ISSUES:
1st row - Hydrogen	**Existence and birth** Has the question of existence or conception. Am I or am I not? Do I exist or do I not exist? Am I conceived or not yet?
2nd row - Lithium	**Separation** Conception happens, the child exists and child grows in the womb. Now it is time to separate. This row signifies this process of separation.
3rd row - Natrum	**Identity** You are now separate and you are out of the womb.

	But do you have an identity yet?
4th row - Calcarea	**Security and task** It has the issue of security. You have your identity but do you have security? Security is in terms of money, relationships, house, job and health.
5th row - Strontium	**Creativity and performance** It is the row of adventure and learning something new.
6th row - Barium	**Responsibility** Taking responsibility for yourself and others.
7th row - Radium	**Disintegration and death**

All the remedies in the Barium row will express the feeling of being handicapped. Aurum and Platina may say I don't want to be handicapped, don't want to be powerless, don't want to be dependent on someone, my worst fear is apprehension.

The remedies in the Calcarea row will have fear of poverty, darkness, robbers, lack of security. It is necessary to see to what extent they have grown out of this and have the ability to counter this situation. The patient may say: "My husband doesn't have an opinion of himself; he takes on the opinion of others. I like to see people who are different, not people like me, but different from me." Then it is an early stage of development, beyond Stage 1 but not Stage 10 yet.

The mineral remedies can be further classified into various groups:

Cations

The main theme of the Cations is the need for a relationship, but this theme gets a characteristic turn in each group.

The theme of Cations of Group IA is forming of relationships (Sodium and Potassium). For Group IIA elements (Magnesium, Calcium, Strontium, Barium, etc.) the theme is a need for support.

Group III elements (Boron and Aluminum) have a feeling of confusion and a sensation as if there was a cobweb on the face.

Anions

The main theme among the Anions is the effort to keep or maintain a relationship.

In Group V (Phosphorus, Arsenicum, Antimonium, Bismuth) the theme is a feeling of being unloved and alone with symptoms like: "Fear of being alone," "Desire for company," "Clinging."

Among the elements of Group VI, (Sulphur and Selenium), the common symptoms are "Aversion to company" and "Incapacity to work." The theme is making an enormous effort which is expected from them.

Group VII contains the halogens (Fluorine, Chlorine, Bromine, Iodine). They have a central feeling of being let down and being betrayed.

Group IV contains the non-metallic elements Carbon and Silica. The feature common to both is that they are non-reactive.

Metals

Among the mineral remedies, the metals have to do with performance and defense. The first line of metals in the Periodic Table is concerned with defense more than performance. This line consists of Manganum, Ferrum, Cobalt, Niccolum, Cuprum and Zincum. The second line has more to do with performance than with defense, and includes Rhodium, Palladium, Argentum, Cadmium and Indium. The elements belonging to the third line have the strongest defense/performance issues. This line consists of the heaviest metals and includes Osmium, Iridium, Platinum, Aurum, Mercury and Thallium.

Thus the degree of defense/performance increases from the first to the third line.

In a mineral case the patient can need an element alone or in combination with some other element as in a salt. In this case it is important to ask the following questions:

- Does one element alone explain the Vital Sensation of the patient completely?
- Does the patient express the theme of more than one element in their Vital Sensation and at the Level of Delusion?

In the case where one element is necessary then it is possible to use Carbonicum as a neutral salt. For example, in a case where Natrum is desired then Natrum carbonicum would be given.

Salts

A salt represents the union of two qualities which balance each other and together are appropriate in certain life situations. Of course the two components of a salt, the Cations and the Anions, need to form a relationship, though they also sometimes seem to repel each other. For example the quality of Natrum is a strong desire to form a relationship, so much so that any rejection can cause tremendous hurt and disappointment. This need of Natrum has to be balanced by a quality of expecting disappointment and rejection, and unwillingness to form relationships. This is provided by the Muriaticum element (Chlorine). Thus, Natrum muriaticum is understandably a very basic salt, for it represents man's need to form relationships and at the same time the ability to withstand rejection.

Acids

The main theme of the acid group is a struggle followed by collapse. The acid of a particular element represents a constant effort/struggle in the situation of that element. For example the main feeling of Phosphorus is that he is unloved and he reacts to this feeling by being affectionate, friendly and sympathetic in the hope that his love and care will be reciprocated. The effort of Phosphorus is therefore in the direction of caring for others, being sympathetic towards them, etc. When this effort becomes constant, i.e., when he feels the need to make a constant effort in caring for others, the state is that of Phosphoricum acidum.

In a state of health the Vital Sensation around the issue of structure diminishes and the healthy person is now able to deal with issues far beyond structure.

G. NOSODES

The theme of nosodes is desperation, which is expressed in every sphere of the life of a person who requires one of these remedies. His way of looking at things and reacting to them is always desperate. Nosodes are prepared from diseased tissue. This tissue is completely under the spell of and overwhelmed by the infection, so that the very basic qualities of the infection or the infectious process manifest in the nosode. In the case of scabies, the tissue will have the qualities of the scabetic infection. The main symptom of scabies is an intense itching. It is a constant struggle with extreme discomfort. The nosode is prepared from the defeated scabies tissue, Psorinum manifests this struggle. The indication for the nosode lies in the process rather than in any particular sphere or area of life. For example, where there is an intense struggle with a problem, be it money, acceptability, religion or love, the indicated remedy is Psorinum. The problem here is of an undifferentiated character. But if the problem is specific to any particular sphere, for example if the struggle has to do with ego and money, the indicated remedy is Sulphur, one of the best known anti-psorics. The nosode thus represents the centerpoint of the miasm.

H. SARCODES AND IMPONDERABLES

Sarcodes and Imponderables are also separate categories to distinguish a remedy choice. There is very little information about these areas at this time. The indication for these remedies will be very clear Source language at the Level of Sensation and Energy.

I. TABLE ON KINGDOMS

Dr. Rajan Sankaran

(This table provides hints to the kingdoms but cannot be used to confirm for certainty without identifying the Vital Sensation and confirming the language of the kingdom at Level 5 Sensation and Level 6 Energy.)

KINGDOM	ANIMAL	MINERAL	PLANT
Features	- Issues of survival - Split - High and low - Victim and aggressor - Strong and weak - Predator and prey - One versus the other - Dominating and dominated - Persecutor and persecuted - Camouflage - Conflict - Split within the self - "I hate myself" - "I am disgusted with myself" - Attractive - Sexual - Instinct to kill - Contradiction of will - Group feeling - Connection to the source	- Structure - Role - Relationship - Performance - Attack and defense - Something is lacking in their identity/relationship /performance/ power - Lack of identity/ support/position/ security/relation/ power - Completeness or incompleteness in self - Fear of losing the completeness	- Basic experience in every area is one common sensation and the opposite - Example: Tight and loose in Euphorbiaceae family, and pain and numbness in Papavaraceae family - Sensitivity and reactivity - Emotional/ sentimental - Disorganized
Talk	- "I will jump at them" - "I will beat them" - "She is better than	- "My relationship" - "My identity" - "My home/family" - "My bank balance"	- "I am affected by" - "I am sensitive to" - "This hurts me" - "This touches me"

KINGDOM	ANIMAL	MINERAL	PLANT
Talk (continued)	me" - "I am not good enough" - "I don't accept myself" - "I feel split up" - "Human beings are so cruel" - Who affects? - Who wins? - Who survives?	- "My health" - "My performance" - "My work" - "My responsibility" - "My joints" - "My skin" - "My nerves"	- "I can't bear this" - "I am immediately affected by"
Signature and Handwriting	- Attention seeking - Aggressive - Attractive - Colorful, esp. for bright colors	- Structured - Angled - Straight	- Rounded - Disorganized
Speech	- Attention seeking - Excited - Animated - Vivid - Moderate to fast-paced	- To the point and finish - Uniform	- All sorts of things that affect them - Varied
Nature and Disposition	- Affectionate - Caring - Playful - Amorous - Aggressive - Mischievous - Alert - Quick to react - Animated - Restless - Deceitful - Curious - Malicious - Jealous - Expressive - Communicative	- Systematic - Strong - Calculative - Organized - Fastidious	- Soft - Sensitive - Emotional - Sentimental - Disorganized - Adjusting - Influenced easily - Adaptable - Irritable
Fears	- Loss in attractiveness - Competition - Aggression - Attack - Rejection - Isolation	- Break of structure (identity/security/performance/power) - Falling of structure - Falling of performance - Losing something	- Hurt - Pain
Dreams and	- Animals	- Structured things	- Nature

KINGDOM	ANIMAL	MINERAL	PLANT
Interests Dreams and Interests (continued)	- Snakes - Pursuit - Attacked - Amorous - Flying	- Financial - Relations - House - Work/effort - Performance - Fight - Repetitive	- Greenery - Plants - Nature - Plants - Artistic - Music - Varied - Influenced by previous days' occurrences
Mode	- Many Faces - Changeable - Abrupt change - Unsteady - Restless	- One mode or two (maximum) - Fixed - Unvarying - Similar in all situations - Steady	- Changeable - Adaptable - Unsteady
Miasmic Range	- Acute to Syco-syphilitic	- Acute to Syphilitic	- Acute to Syphilitic
Key word	- Competition	- Structure	- Sensitivity
Manner of Dressing	- Attractive or dull - Unusual - Animals in dress (snake rings, etc.)	- Patterns - Checks - Structured - Plain - Symmetry	- Flowery - Sensitive - Irregular patterns
Profession	- Advertising - Competitions	- Accounting - Computers - Management - House builders - Engineers - Performers	- Artists - Nurses
Complaint Presentation	- With feeling - Animated - Attention seeking - Warm - Alert eyes - Eye contact	- Organized - Structured - Percentages - Systematic - Written points - Exactness - Numbers	- Haywire - Rounded - Wandering - Descriptive - Adjusting - Symptoms described randomly and not completely
Nature of Complaint	- Problems in attractiveness and competitiveness	- Problems in structure - Chronic	- Sensitivity - Many modalities - Influenced easily - Quick reaction
Pace	- Generally moderate to fast paced	- Generally slow onset and progress	- Generally rapid onset and variations
Causation	- Rejection	- Break of structure	- Emotional or

KINGDOM	ANIMAL	MINERAL	PLANT
Causation (continued)	- Neglect - Looked down on - Failure in defense - Failure in competition - Aggression/attack - Failure in love	- Break of relationship - Failure in performance - Failure in power/ responsibility	physical hurt - Shock/strain

I. SAMPLE CASES

By Melissa Burch, CCH

CASE 1

CASE of YOUNG MAN with FATIGUE	ANALYSIS
Homeopath: Alright, so what is the problem going on with you?	
Client: Okay, right this moment, I've had boils around my toes. This is a problem that I've had over the last two or three years, about once a year. I'm actually grateful when they appear around my toes as opposed to previous times they were on the soles of my feet, which meant I absolutely couldn't even walk. But these boils are recurring. In previous years, I have sought treatment at a local health center. These treatments seemed to help, but now the boils are coming back again. So that is the main impetus for why I am here. There are also other, more chronic, ongoing things that I suffer from. Like I also have tiredness and low energy (compared to how I used to be). Those would be the two main additional things.	
Those are the two main things, okay. And of those two, which one is the more…	*Looking for the Chief Complaint.*
The tiredness I would say, well, the tiredness is clearly a chronic thing, and it feels the most acute. Also on an acute level, I get herpes occasionally, but that comes and goes.	
Where at?	

CASE of YOUNG MAN with FATIGUE	**ANALYSIS**
Around the genitals. And that's…I find the herpes comes more from…I don't know…the closest I can get is almost like Christian guilt. It feels like when my partner and I are physically intimate together, and if we are really close on an energetic level, then I generally don't get the herpes. Whereas if it starts to become more like sex than making love, if I block out (*HG*) and am just sort of off, then I can often get herpes soon after that. So that's the ongoing thing. But it's usually confined to a sexual context, whereas with the boils, I'm not sure why I get them. I have the belief that when I used to live in another city, and although I walked around barefoot a lot, I never had any problems. But when I moved to this new city (where I live now), I was walking around barefoot and I got, in the spring, these really bad boils. And I don't know. Some people said it's because of whatever is in the ground, in the earth; it is coming up into my feet. But that's more of an external reason for why I have been afflicted with boils. After a couple of years, though, I started to make sure that I was always wearing sandals, and I didn't get the boils then for quite a long time. But it's interesting that recently, in the monsoon, we were doing some gardening and the earth was extremely wet so I took off my shoes, just for a half an hour, because they were getting stuck in the mud. And then one or two days later I got the boils on my toes. I've been trying to look at it from other angles, whether it's this or it's that, whether it's making steps in life, anger, whatever. And it's not been easy between my partner and me in the last weeks, either, months. It's been an up and down thing *(HG up and down)*, so I don't know if the boils have something to do with that. But then I feel we've also made quite some steps. So if that was the reason behind it, considering the steps we've made in the last weeks, I feel that it would have cleared up fairly quickly. So I was wondering if there was some other internal process (*HG circles*) going on which triggered the boils to come.	*Story………….* *(HG) is strong hand gesture* *Story…………*

CASE of YOUNG MAN with FATIGUE	ANALYSIS
Can you talk about the boils a bit, what they feel like, what's the…	*Still looking for the Chief Complaint.*
They are extremely annoying. They are usually only painful before they appear. There's this volcanic feeling, this build-up of pressure and pain under the surface of my skin. And if there is some pain there, I know that in a day or two there will be a boil there. But you wouldn't actually even see anything there…it's just this build up, almost like a tingly sensation mixed with pain and then it starts throbbing.	*Fact Level with Local Sensation and Delusion.* *Local Sensation.*
You said it's almost volcanic, as the pressure is building up.	*Repeat back the Local Sensation and urge the client for more…………*
Yes. It feels on a bodily level how I would almost imagine a volcano feels before it's about to explode. It's just this kind of (rumbling noise) under the surface of the skin and then, of course, it doesn't erupt out in that sense, but it definitely has that sensation. I often have the image of a volcano when I am going through this experience.	*Delusion with Energy……*
So tell me more about this volcanic experience that you're going through.	*Ask about the Experience of the Image – Not the Image/Volcano itself.*
Well, it's like the body is drawing the pus, or whatever is in the boil, to the toes, or whatever place. And it's picking that place to build up and build up and build up and when there's enough there, then there's that eruption, as a boil.	*Local Sensation*
And this pain, this pressure, can you describe it a little bit more, this pain, before this…	
It's really, it's like this throbbing, like a deep	*Local Sensation – Not progressing beyond the Local. Not so*

CASE of YOUNG MAN with FATIGUE	**ANALYSIS**
throbbing pain.	*much Energy. No sign of a Vital Expression. Do we have the Chief Complaint with the Most Energy?*
So of all these things, again, what would be to you the most problematic, the boils, the herpes, the tiredness?	
The boils, the boils don't, I mean, they're annoying, but they don't bother me so much. And I can't say they affect my life in a day to day way. The herpes can really get in the way of my relationship, so that definitely affects me. And on another level, the tiredness, yes. I'd say the tiredness somehow has more of a profound effect on me. For example, the children will go to bed at 9 o'clock and my partner will be looking forward to having a couple of hours, just the two of us. Then by half past nine I'm ready for bed, almost to the point where I can't keep my eyes open. We'll be having a conversation, and it's clear to me that if it's a deeper conversation and it starts to touch issues in me, then it's like there's a light-switch inside me that goes, "click." (*Strong HG indicating and sound)* and she sees this in me too certain topics might come up and I might really be nodding. I will have to almost hold my eyes open. It's like an internal defense mechanism.	*Let's follow this as a Chief Complaint.* *Experience of the Chief Complaint in Delusion Language.* *Possible Vital Expression because of the Strong Energy of the Expression.* *Listening for the Vital Expression............*
You said it's like a light-switch.	
Yes, I said it's like a switch. (*HG a bit similar to the "block out" gesture*) Like the body or the mind or the ego or whatever just goes, "uh-oh—click—let's press the tiredness escape button." (*Big HG*) And off I go. So yes, I have a feeling that if the switch wasn't there, and if I could be more present and energized (*HG – two hands at chest*) in a regular way, I would…yeah, that would help me the most.	*Delusion Language with Energy and Hand Gestures.* *Listen to See if this Idea is confirmed as Vital Expression since it has so much Energy – this "Switch" idea is similar to his earlier reference to "Block Out" and "just sort of off."* *Need More Confirmation.*

CASE of YOUNG MAN with FATIGUE	**ANALYSIS**
Energized…like?	*Following the Non Human Specific/ universal Language accompanied by a Gesture – still listening for a solid Vital Expression...*
Energized. Like having energy, like empowered, like, you know, embodied more. I'm very much in my head. And I do try to do sports and other things…yoga, running, whatever, but I'm very bad at regular activity. I'm very bad at daily anything.	
What do you mean by bad at daily…?	
Like if I have to do a daily meditation practice, or if I have to get up and run every morning, or if I have to cook every night, or if I was always washing dishes every day. I don't have anything against any of those things and I'll happily do all of them irregularly, *(HG)* but I have a real difficulty in doing the same thing, at the same time, everyday. And I don't know how much that has to do with my lack of energy. My partner always mentions things like, if I was doing more sports, if I ran more regularly, or if I was in my body more, that this would help me. And I have no doubt that it would help. In previous times in my life, in my early twenties, I was much more connected to those aspects of my being—the vital—a positive sense of vital energy *(HG)* and of being able to do a lot.	*Story and Situation..........*
Okay, so it's somehow, it's this light-switch and also with the herpes there is some kind of block that comes sometimes.	*The Homeopath comes back to the "light switch" and "I go off" to what the client mentioned earlier regarding the herpes "block out" and "just sort of off."* *Checking for confirmation that these are the same thing in two different areas of his life...*
The herpes I would say is more if I go into my head	

CASE of YOUNG MAN with FATIGUE	**ANALYSIS**
rather than being there with my partner. If we really explore, experiment, and try to forge a connection strongly between us, and if I stay present in that, (*HG*) then everything is fine. Whereas, somehow, if I'm not present, if I don't stay present, then the herpes usually comes one or two days later.	
So what does this staying present for you…I guess your partner talked to you a little bit about what to expect from a homeopathic interview, so you have the sense that I'm going to ask the same questions over and over and over?	*His answer to "block out" and "switch off" has to do with being present – either in conversation about issues or in his sexual relationship regarding intimacy.* *He is making a connection……….*
Okay. Fine.	
I'm going to try to understand it more and more deeply even though you've explained it very well so far and I understand the situation and how it works for you.	*The Homeopath explains the process for encouragement.*
Okay.	
But I'm just going to go more. So staying present, what does that mean, how do you experience that…?	
For me, staying present is really focusing (*HG*) on the bodily feelings, on my emotions, on the connection to her on an energetic level, and being aware of what's going on, of where I am, where she is, and the energy-flow between us. Whereas if I get too stuck in just focusing on my sensations, that for me is not…it's not being present. It's present in a specific way, but when I say being present, I mean in a wider sense (HG).	*Story and Situation………. Hints of Local Sensation.*
Wider sense, what do you mean by a wider	*Following the Hand Gestures.*

CASE of YOUNG MAN with FATIGUE	ANALYSIS
sense?	
Wider in the sense of not just sensations. Not just my sensations, but her sensations too. And like I said, the energy-flow between us—the heart connection. Yes. I'd say maybe I could simply say, focusing on us rather than on me. That would be one way of putting it.	
And then it's also somehow with this light-switch, there is something there when you're in a deep conversation and you're being present, you said, and then it's like the switch goes off. There's somehow…can you relate the two? I'm not clear. Because there too you said that if you're in a deep conversation that it touches something, then the light-switch…	*Going back to what could possibly be a Vital Expression... they had similar gestures. These may mean the same things – the block out and the light switch. We need him to confirm it.*
Yes, but I don't feel the sense of light-switch if my partner and I are physically intimate together. It's kind of more, like I might drift into just my own sensations. But then I have either pulled myself back into the present, into the us, or she draws me back to the us. Then it's all fine. It's not like once I'm gone, then I'm gone, and I can't get back to that. But, for me, the sense of the switch with the tiredness is more that once the switch is gone, I can't…it's like it's out of my control. I can't. No matter how much will power I exert in coming back and wanting to stay present, if there's something inside me that's trying to switch, to shut me down from looking at something I don't want to see, for instance, if that's what it is, the switch will go off. I can sit there and say, "but I want to talk about this, I want to go deeper, I want to understand what's going on inside me, I want to be aware of anything that is trying to emerge and come up into my awareness," but I feel like I'm not in control. And that's a totally different subject, the question of control. But if the switch goes, for example, it's like	*Not quite the same but similar – the "light switch" is more intense then the "block out."*

CASE of YOUNG MAN with FATIGUE	ANALYSIS
it's because my ego, a part of my being which is in control, doesn't want this other part to come up. And it presses the panic button, (*HG indicates*) which is what I referred to as the light-switch. And then suddenly, whoooooof, (*Sound/Energy*) I'm falling asleep. And I can't stop it. I could take cold showers, I could…I even went for a 2-mile-run at midnight once. I was trying to keep awake because my partner and I were having a very intense exchange which I wanted to be present for, but I kept falling asleep. So I went running around the whole community, for two miles, and came back and then fell asleep. So the running didn't help.	
So what it this panic button? It's like a panic button gets pressed and then you fall asleep? Can you describe everything about this panic button?	*Vital Expression is coming together as this Process which includes Block Out, I'm Off, Drift Off, Shut Me Down, Panic Button, plus the Strong Gesture and the Click and Whooof.* *Not Exactly the Same – but the Similar Idea expressed in Two Different Ideas at Two Different Paces.*
That's somehow the closest I can come to describe it. It's taken me awhile to feel that it comes from the sense that there are different parts of my being vying for attention and control, that the one which has the upper hand is kind of pushing down (*Vivid HG*), like it doesn't want another part to emerge. It could be my mental. It could be in my mind. Like I've said, I'm so strongly in my mind.	*Sounds like Animal Language -- "different parts," "upper hand."* *Repeat back the Strong Gesture and All Language and ask him to Tell More about this Experience.* *Listen Not JUST for the WORDS THEMSELVES but the PHENOMENON he is TRYING to DESCRIBE with these WORDS.*
This pushing down, this something is…you show something like this (HG).	
Yes, part of my being, is, let's say, for want of a better word, in control. (*Explaining the HG*) And	*This part is pushing down and this part is trying to come up.*

CASE of YOUNG MAN with FATIGUE	ANALYSIS
then there's this other part of my being, whether it's connecting to my emotions or whatever it might be, that's trying to come up. My sense is that the in-control part of myself feels that it has something to lose, or that it might not be in control anymore, if the other parts are allowed to emerge. So then the in-control part pushes down the panic button because it knows that if it pushes the panic button, then I can't be present anymore to let the emergence of these other parts of my being come through.	*The in-control part is pushing down the coming up parts so that these coming up parts can't be present.* *What is he describing? He is describing how this "panic button" prevents parts of him from Existing.* *He is talking about how part of him is denied and he can't Exist Fully – This is MINERAL KINGDOM.* *The ANIMAL EXPERIENCE is Not Here – it is NOT about MY SURVIVAL and I need to OVERPOWER it or that I am the WEAKER and VICTIM.*
You're explaining it very well, actually. It's quite good, I think. But just a bit more. So somehow there is something that's pressing down and then this other part is coming up and you said it's like this emergence coming through. Just a bit more, of just that experience for you. What do you know about it? Just a few more words.	*Have him flesh this idea out more – Repeat Back the Words and Gestures.*
Hmmm. I'm trying to feel back into a time when it happened. It comes when we're talking about something important. Then I feel that there are blocks to my awareness or my being where I feel I could learn something and grow from it or evolve in some way. It's like if the conversation starts to feel like if it's going in a direction and I can feel there is something just outside of my reach. (*HG*) Like when you have a word on the tip of your tongue and can't quite get it, and you're thinking, "what's that word, what's that word," and you can't quite get it. It's like there's this awareness just out of my reach, and I can't say what it could be because I've not had it before, necessarily, but it almost feels like something from my past or something that could radically change me. Like the sense of an ah-ha moment. Like, "ahh (*HG*) that's why I'm like this	*"Blocks" -- part the Vital Expression Spontaneously Resurface – Good Confirmation we are on the Right Track.* *Now he goes back to Story and Situation and looses the Non Human Specific Language.*

CASE of YOUNG MAN with FATIGUE	ANALYSIS
or that's why I do this," or, 'that's why, I react in such and such a way to this type of a situation." And so there's a part of me that really yearns for that understanding, that yearns for those moments when I can really feel, "oh, okay, so that happened in my childhood and therefore maybe that's why I act like this and maybe I can change it, then maybe I don't have to feel controlled or under the sway of this past event." I want to be as clear in my being as possible, to respond from a clear place in my being and not just robotically (HG). You know, that's how I respond if I'm afraid, or if I'm angry, or whatever it may be. So it's that sense that there's something just out of reach.	
It's just out of reach?	*What does this mean for him? Listening for More Confirmation of the Kingdom.*
Somehow, yes. It usually happens if I'm having a conversation with my partner. It can happen if we go to bed and she's hoping we'll make love, but I go to sleep. And it's not because I don't want to make love to her. There's something there also that can happen (*HG – Hand moves down across body – similar Direction and Energy of earlier Gesture*) where it's just this…	
The something that also comes, what's this (HG)?	*What is "this" with the Gesture?*
That's this sense of black. Well, blackness that comes from tiredness that comes from the closing of the eyes and the body switching off. It's just this shut off (*HG – similar to earlier Gestures – Strong and Repeated throughout this conversation*). So that's why I sense a light-switch. This switching off, this darkness (*HG*), maybe that's why I used light-switch because the switch is going off, not going on, and then the darkness that comes from that. And the darkness is also connected to ignorance. Ignorance about myself. But also, I have this wanting to	*Okay – Now we have a Solid Confirmation that our Vital Expression is indeed this "Switch Off", "Shut Off," etc.....* *We are On Solid Ground. Now we just need to Pursue his Experience of the Vital Expression Fully to Understand and Confirm the Kingdom.* *He is talking at All Levels Now – Delusion, Situation, Emotional, Energy, ...* *This discussion of Parts hints at Mineral.*

CASE of YOUNG MAN with FATIGUE	ANALYSIS
know, wanting to understand what makes me tick in different ways. And in a sense I'm getting close, but there's this part of my being that is getting in the way. It says, "uh-uh, you're not ready for that one yet (*HG -- Fingers*)." Or this part of me doesn't want to know about that yet.	*Listen that it is not Parts in Battle for Survival as Much as it is Parts that are Missing or Not Allowed to Express themselves so he can fully be Present/Exist.* *Issues about Understanding Myself -- 3rd Row Issues of Identity. I am here but who am I.*
This part of me, what is that, this (HG-fingers)?	
This is me trying to represent different parts of my being whether it's in this shoulder or this shoulder or whether it's up here or…	*Following the New Gesture.*
Right, right, but what is this, what do you think, just this (HG), this part of you that's (HG) like this, what is this? Just that?	
It's fuzzy, it's not clear. It's…this is (*HG Fingers*) fuzziness.	*Moving in Source Language – Quality Words.....*
Fuzziness? What does fuzziness mean?	
Lack of clarity. It's like hazy, it's like wanting, foggy, misty, opaque. (*Lots of Gestures*) It's on the other side, but I'd like to see it, and I'd like to be made aware of it. If I go like this (*HG*), or if I'm saying it's hazy like this (*HG*), that's more between me and something else out there. The reason I went like this (*HG*) is because it's in me. I feel like it's all inside me. It's in here (*HG to head*), or wherever. I'm not seeing it as an external thing so much. It's an internal sense, like a hazy area of myself. It's like there's a part of me that I can't connect to.	*Source Words coming up.* *He is Differentiating Kingdom Beautifully here....* *He Differentiates that it is Not Animal (Victim/Aggressor) but Mineral (about Parts of his Existence). He has All the Parts – just can't connect to some of them.*

<u>**CASE of YOUNG MAN with FATIGUE**</u>	<u>**ANALYSIS**</u>
Good. Everything about this hazy part of yourself that you cannot connect to…you've explained it very well and the circumstances that it comes up under. But just as much as you can say about that hazy part of you that doesn't connect…	*Focus on the Source Words Now......*
(Long pause)	
You can do that again (HG), it's quite helpful sometimes. This hazy part of you, you said it's foggy, it's misty, it stops you from doing…you'd like to be aware—it stops you from being aware…	*Encourage him to Use the Gesture to go Deeper.*
It' a good question, I mean, it's kind of like on the one side, I've put a lot of trust in my mental capacities. I see that my mental has got me through life—that's my inner belief, I'm sure it's not true, but it's my inner belief. Like at school I've never done a sport, but my head has somehow got me through and…	*Going into Situation and Emotion but LISTEN for SOURCE WORDS NOW as well as information to help us confirm the ROW, SIDE of the PERIODIC TABLE and ultimately the COLUMN.* *He is telling us is he has Full Mental Capacity – he is Not Trying to Get this – he has it. He has ALL the PARTS. The problem is he "switches off" and can't connect to certain parts...* *This tells us he is RIGHT of CENTER on the Periodic Table.*
So it's your mental capacity that got you through?	
Somehow, yes.	
What do you mean by mental capacity in this sense?	

CASE of YOUNG MAN with FATIGUE	**ANALYSIS**
Well, I should say mental as opposed to my physical or emotional.	
But just what does mental capacity mean for you? If I didn't speak English or didn't know what those words meant, can you then talk about it?	*Make them Define their Words.*
Being able to talk well, being able to understand things quickly, being able to communicate, having quite a vivid imagination. As an architect, it helps…	*For him Mental Capacity is about his IDENTITY – being able to Talk, Understand, Communicate.* *ROW THREE*
Well, how does that relate then to this hazy feeling? It doesn't connect to something that you want to be aware of.	
Yes, the reason I mention this is because I feel I'm trying to contrast it in the sense that I like to understand things, I like to be clear, I like clarity. I don't like fuzziness. I can live with a certain fuzziness, but if I can make it clearer, I prefer that. I want to be able to understand things. So I think my sense of this (*HG Fingers*) is representative of those parts of myself that I don't understand very well. I'd like to defuzzify (*HG Fingers*) them and get the fuzz out. I'd like to make the opaque glass transparent so I can see through and go "ahh," this sense of, "I do this because that happened back then, or I do this for whatever reason." So I can explain the fuzziness by contrasting it in that way.	*Source Words – Fuzzy, Opaque, Transparent...* *Mixture of Situation and Delusion.* *All of this is How can he be Him – have an IDENTITY. He is already HERE (Row 1 and 2). For him it is about how he can fully be himself.* *Has the Parts of Himself – he knows THEY are THERE but he can't seem to connect to them – something to do with the past.*
Yes, that's good. Go ahead and describe it as much in the contrast, more, it's something not clear, to make the opaque glass transparent…	*Repeat back Source Words........*
My sense is because I've relied on my mental capacities to get me through life, to some degree or	*Delusion Language but Listen for SOURCE and ROW/COLUMN LANGUAGE.*

CASE of YOUNG MAN with FATIGUE	**ANALYSIS**
another, that there's a part of my ego connected strongly to that. And I believe that there's a part of my ego that doesn't want my emotional side, or my vital side, to have more say or to be more present. That's why I said earlier that it's as if my ego is pushing the panic button.	*Aspect of Vital Expression reappears – Great Confirmation!*
What is ego for you? What is this ego that's pushing this panic button? What is that?	*Ask again about this Aspect of the Vital Expression to urge him deeper.*
I think for me the ego is kind of my sense of self that I've created over the years. You know, David the architect, David the Englishman, David the whatever. I don't know. Whatever my picture of myself is, this is for me the ego. And I think so much of that construct has clarity, and I'm quite happily attached to that in many ways. But those are the parts of me that I'd like to explore. Like I said, my mental got me so far, and I'm sure my mental could keep me going for many years to come, quite happily. But that's not what I'm here for. I want to explore these other parts of my being. I want to understand what makes me tick in other ways.	*Story and Delusion but this is where we get Row Information for the Periodic Table.* *Clearly ROW THREE/IDENTITY – "I am David the Englishman," "I am David the Architect."* *He has a FULLY FORMED IDENTITY – the problem is lost connection with part of it. This Pushes us to the RIGHT SIDE of the PERIODIC TABLE.*
What makes you tick, what do you mean by makes you tick?	
What makes me who I am that isn't just my mental, the, "hi I'm David I'm an architect," like, "hi I'm David I'm a human being." At times, I would like not to have these mental labels, just to explore, because the label can be just as much an imprisonment as it can be a help.	*This is All about IDENTITY.* *Issue with Labels – being Defined One Way. This can be Imprisonment.*
As a what?	
As a help. Like a label can help to understand	*Delusion and Story......*

CASE of YOUNG MAN with FATIGUE	**ANALYSIS**
<u>somebody, but it can also, "oh, David's an architect, we put him in the architect box."</u> <u>That means you can't be something else necessarily</u>. And although that's a kind of basic example, I think it works on many, many levels and in more subtle ways. <u>It's an easy example for me, that if I tell you I'm an architect, then you think of me as an architect. Whereas for me, inside myself, this is where I keep trying to get back to what makes me like I am</u>. Is it from a previous experience in my childhood? Is it from some chemical imbalance in my body? <u>I don't know, whatever it might be I am interested in getting closer to the real me, and when I say the real me I mean not just this mental construct of "this is who I am</u>." And that's where the ego comes in because <u>I think the ego is strengthened, or created even, through all my mental constructs</u>, over all of the years of my life to build up to, "<u>David is this.</u>"	*I don't want this LABEL -- I want to be who I am!* *Delusional Ideas that fit a Particular Third Row Remedy..........* *His Issue is I have this Label – I built this Label of "David" but maybe I am or want to be something else – Not this.* *This is the Delusional Situation of CHLORUM from Scholten.*
And this is what presses the panic button?	*Seeking Clarification.*
Somehow I feel that, yes.	
This, you said, construct?	
Yes. The ego…	
You're doing great, actually. I'm really understanding it very well. You're actually quite clear. It's not that, it's just trying to put it together so it's actually very clear. We're just trying to understand more the dimension, because it's actually quite multi-dimensional. What you're trying to explain involves multiple layers: this construct that needs to be in control; then somehow it presses the panic button; and the light; the switch goes off; and then it's the darkness. So it's just trying to understand the whole, all of the angles. So the ego, you said, is	*Explaining where you are in the case to the client and where you want to go.*

CASE of YOUNG MAN with FATIGUE	**ANALYSIS**
this mental construct, is this for you the main theme? Are we on the right direction? Is that something that's really been…?	
Yes, I think so.	
It sounds like it. It sounds like this is where this starts from.	
It's the closest I can get to it I would say, yes.	
So what is the mental construct then? More about that…this mental construct that is you, that you identify as David-the-architect and then it's in the box, just more…	*Define more Terms.*
Well, a mental construct can be anything. One example, though, would be how I choose to portray myself. Like, do I wear a shirt like this, or do I wear a plaid shirt? Do I walk around in shoes, or do I walk around in sandals? It's sort of like 36 years of conditioning…by society, by peers, by parents. The mind understands that as a child in the playground, if you look like this, you'll get picked on; if you look like that, you won't. It's a mental construct that goes into my understanding, my mental understanding, that informs me to decide whether I want to get picked on or not, or how I want to be in society, with people around me. Mental constructs are the images that we build up around ourselves. Our story, you know. Where I came from, what makes me who I am, whatever it may be. So yes, I can sit here and analyze the past (I probably think quite often about the past). I think I often rationalize my present state and where I am going. I look for patterns. I see, "okay, I came from here, and I've done this, and here I am now." So this movement now makes sense. That's what I mean by mental construct, that I'm looking for this	*Am I this? OR am I that?* *Delusion and Story.* *All about Him and Who he is in the World.*

CASE of YOUNG MAN with FATIGUE	**ANALYSIS**
understanding, this explanation, for an action or a way of being.	
Yes, it's like a movement, like you use it to see a movement. What is your understanding of this movement?	*Picking out the Non Human Specific word from the Story.*
Movement in life, it's where I'm going, it's why I'm here. And I think I probably seek to understand the movement because my mental still has a very strong place in my being. I'm still using it to rationalize, on some level, my actions or my way of being. On the other hand, there are things I feel in my heart. For example, my heart feels right that I'm here in this place in my life, and it knows it doesn't want to be anywhere else. But that's not enough. Well…it should be enough. I'd like to just have it fit quite happily. I'd like to know that if my heart tells me I'm in the right place, that it should somehow be enough. But why do I need to sit around thinking every now and then, or however often, that, "okay, I'm here, this is why I'm here and this is what I'm doing, and it makes sense doing what I'm doing, and it's doing me good (whatever that might mean), good for my spiritual growth, good for…you know, I'm doing what I came on this planet to do." And if I'm not doing what I should do, at least I'm doing something positive and not making more of a mess of the world.	*More Story and Delusion.*
But you said you should be in the right place…it should be enough, to be in the right place. What does being in the right place mean for you?	*Trolling for more info.*
Being in the right place, for many years of my life, simply meant where my head told me I should be. But what I'd like it to mean is where my heart feels it should be. And I think at the moment, I have	*In terms of what Level he Lives on in a Day to Day Life – Mostly Delusion – he does not seem to be able to access his Emotions.*

CASE of YOUNG MAN with FATIGUE	ANALYSIS
both. At the moment, my heart and my head are quite happily content to be where I am, doing what I am doing. But I would like to explore further into myself…more into my heart, into my emotions. I have been, in the past, quite a cool person. This statement is partly based on other people's experience of me, the feedback I've received occasionally over the years. But also, even just in myself, I agree…I am not very extroverted emotionally. And I say emotionally, because I can be quite extroverted non-emotionally. Meaning, I can sit at a table at a dinner party and be just as much a part of the conversation as everyone else (not necessarily the life and soul of the party) but holding my own. And again, maybe it is on an intellectual level, but it's the whole, on a mental level, knowing that, "I can act like this, and this is what you get in life." Like when you take various cultural inputs over the years, whether it's watching a film, being with friends, or reading a book, and it forms a mental map: if you want to be funny, you do this; if you want to be successful at architecture, you do that.	
But somehow this construct, this ego you called it, that's the thing that presses the panic button, which is somehow connected to, you said, to the heart, or the emotions, or something in the past maybe, that you're trying to understand. Can we just go back to that one more time? Just what that experience is like, not so much for you, because you've described it very well, but if you just had to describe to someone, like if you put yourself aside and just describe what that would be like for…I know it's a little difficult but if you just…	*Trying to Dissociate him from his Story and Get back to Sensation Level and urge him Towards Source.*
When you say not as me…?	
Yes, because now you've explained very well:	

CASE of YOUNG MAN with FATIGUE	**ANALYSIS**
you, for who you are, and for you to have had a mental construct of yourself. You've been very successful in that. You've painted quite a good picture of that. And somehow it's the thing that presses this panic button, is that right?	
That's my sense of it, yes. That's as close as I can come to it.	
Yes, it is very clear, and it's actually quite good. So just more, if you could just talk about what that experience is like, not so much from your situation, but just what that action might be like of pressing the panic button.	*Going back to an aspect of the Vital Expression and bring back to Kingdom.*
This action, you mean the action of this part of my being, how that part acts?	
Or just what it would be like to press a panic button in another situation. You can be quite free now, or open, whatever comes to mind. What is it like to have something pressing a panic button that makes you immediately tired and you have to go to sleep? You've explained very well how it all works. Just take it one more step to separate from you to what this action is like, how you might describe that to someone who's not so much in your situation. Because you've done a very good job of describing your own particular situation, but just what is that action of something that presses a panic button and then has to go into the blackness?	DISSOCIATE.
And when you ask about the action, do you mean I should actually describe it, is it like this, is it like this?	
Whatever comes to mind and how you can	

CASE of YOUNG MAN with FATIGUE	ANALYSIS
relate to it. You've done a good job at the circumstances and the understanding of how it fits you, and now I just want to abstract it out a little bit.	
Okay, so I think the actual definition of the pressing a panic button or clicking the light-switch, if I feel into the action more concretely, is actually like a fog rising up around me. (*HG*) It's like I'm sitting there and looking around and wanting to look more around, and then this feeling, this…is it a feeling? It's a feeling in the sense of the tiredness, but it's more that this fog just lifts and rises around me and then…a kind of loss of control.	*Listening Now for SOURCE LANGUAGE.* *Fog Rising Up, Rises............ Ties into the Chief Complaint!*
Great, so tell me more about the qualities of this fog, it rises up and then you…?	*Looking for SOURCE which is going to be QUALITY WORDS.*
Long Pause.........................It's dense, it's has a heaviness. Pause................ it's almost, the word that comes to mind is embodied ignorance. It's like ignorance in matter. This fog is tangible, (*HG -- grabbing*) like (cotton candy), the stuff you get at fairs in big pink balls. The fog is not pink, but it's tangible in the sense that you could actually put your hand around it. It seems almost physical, like you can put your hand through it (*HG*). On the verge of being tangible, it feels like you can grab it.	*You can see him going inwards........* *Lots of Gestures – Energy.*
It's almost on the verge of being tangible, and it has what kind of qualities?	
There's this denseness, this heaviness, this…	
Denseness, heaviness, some more words…	
Thick. Clammy. Yeah, it's kind of clammy.	

CASE of YOUNG MAN with FATIGUE	**ANALYSIS**
Does it feel moist?	
Yes, and then I have this image, as the fog is rising, it functions like a drug. I feel drugged when I get this tiredness. Like I feel drugged – whooff I'm gone. It really feels like I could have just had a shot in the arm, and then it's like…I'm gone. It is like if I imagine a tear gas or some kind of gas that creates an effect. It's like this fog rising has the effect of anesthesia, like I'm just out of the count completely.	*Again reconnects to the Chief Complaint.* *Bringing back earlier language – connecting it all together for you.* *Delusion at Source Level – Listen to the Qualities.*
And the tear gas, and the anesthesia, a little bit more about what you know about those substances.	*Check Named Sources but Listening for what DOESN'T FIT.*
The only reason I use tear gas is because it's used against people. Because this gas rises (*HG*) and people have the reaction of crying and swelling eyes. I've never experienced it myself personally, but I use it as a metaphor more than the shot in the arm because when I feel it, it's coming like a fog. (*HG*) I feel the fog has something quite strongly to do with this tiredness. It's like there could be some chemical reaction going on with this fog around me, where that makes me fall to sleep. Like a sleeping gas or something like that. I see it as an externally manifested thing that I can hold, rather than just something going on inside me. It's like being injected with some kind of drug that puts me to sleep.	*It is Not Tear Gas.*
Right, you are very clear. Can you tell me about your dreams?	
Hmmm, I knew you were going to ask me that…one of the strongest dreams I ever had was when my partner and I both woke up on the same	

CASE of YOUNG MAN with FATIGUE	ANALYSIS
night with the same dream. We were in a native tribe and somebody died and the people thought I did it. But I hadn't done it, so I chose to run away. I felt I had to leave the tribe. The strongest part of the dream was when I was running through the forest, being chased by the tribe's people, and I ending up in a forest clearing. I was so tired and exhausted that I just collapsed right in the middle of the clearing. In that moment, I knew it was done because they were just behind me. And when they came into the clearing, I died.	*Connects to the Chief Complaint.*
What was this feeling that you were running through this forest in this dream, they were chasing you, and then you said you felt so tired and exhausted you collapsed? Do you remember what that sensation was like, of running and knowing they were right there and then you were so exhausted?	
Knowing what the sensation of being exhausted was like?	
Well, you described that you were running and they were chasing you, and then something happened where all of the sudden you felt so tired…	
No, I was tired already, I mean, I was running and running and running. And I was already tired and somehow, for whatever reason, the place where I actually collapsed or fell or tripped or whatever, was this clearing in the forest. And maybe I just decided that was the place I was going to die. That was it. It was there…the rain, the moon. It was the moment. And from the dream I don't remember being afraid, it was more like, "okay, this is it—so be it."	

CASE of YOUNG MAN with FATIGUE	ANALYSIS
That's my memory. That's what I carry in me now from that dream, but I wonder…	Remedy: Chlorum Potency: 200C

ADDITIONAL NOTES: Remedy is Chlorum, not Chloroform. Chlorum is used in Anesthesia; Chloroform has a carbon element, and we are not seeing a carbon theme here.

Background: Had stopped having a relationship with his Mother. She would always chase him around when he visited her – drove him nuts so cut off relationship with her.

After remedy: Boils and allergies came and went. Then the memory of being sexually molested by his grandfather returned. This was this "fuzzy thing" that he couldn't understand himself. Then he realized he rejected his mother, not that she rejected him. He did the rejecting, as he doesn't want to be told what his Identity is. He has since re-established a relationship with his mother.

Chlorum has all these issues around the relationship with the mother, fleeing from the relationship with the mother on the delusional level.

Understanding the remedy along the columns of the 3rd row of the periodic table:

Phosphorus has the theme of "friends and identity". The client did not display this as his issue.

Sulfur is about "identity through ideas, through relationship". The client did not display this idea of "one partner makes me whole".

Chlorum is two-and-a-half times thicker than air, and is the most abundant ion in salt water.

Overview: Quite loquacious; self-, ego-, identity- focused client. Sounded a bit Animal Kingdom because talks about different parts in himself, but more about the parts he needs to fully exist (Mineral Kingdom), not parts in competition for survival (Animal Kingdom).

Chief Complaint: fatigue

Vital Expression: block out, switch off, shut off

Some questions homeopath asks, once VE is identified:

Okay, so it's somehow, it's this light-switch and also with the herpes there is some kind of block that comes sometimes. Use the word block.

So what is this panic button? It's like a panic button gets pressed and then you fall asleep? Can you describe everything about this panic button?

This pushing down, this something is...you show something like this (HG)?

You're explaining it very well, actually. But just a bit more. So somehow there is something that's pressing down and then this other part is coming up and you said it's like this emergence coming through? Just a bit more, of just that experience for you.

The something that also comes, what's this (HG)?

Good. Everything about this hazy part of yourself that you cannot connect to... You can do that again (HG), it's quite helpful sometimes. This hazy part of you, you said it's foggy, it's misty, it stops you from doing...you'd like to be aware—it stops you from being aware...

But just what does mental capacity mean for you? If I didn't speak English or didn't know what those words meant, can you then talk about it?

What is ego for you? What is this ego that's pushing this panic button? What is that?

If you could just talk about what that experience is like, not so much from your situation, but just what that action might be like of pressing the panic button. Or just what it would be like to press a panic button in another situation. You can be quite free now, or open, whatever comes to mind. What is it like to have something pressing a panic button that makes you immediately tired and you have to go to sleep? *(trying to dissociate client)*

Kingdom and Sub-kingdom Language: Mineral Kingdom, 3rd Row of Periodic Table

My sense is that the in-control part of myself feels that it has something to lose, or that it might not be in control anymore, if the other parts are allowed to emerge. So then the in-control part pushes down the panic button because it knows that if it pushes the panic button, then I can't be present anymore to let the emergence of these other parts of my being come through. *(This could sound a bit Animal Kingdom, but because it is more about existing fully, and not about survival, it is Mineral Kingdom.)*

There's this part of my being that is getting in the way. It says, "Uh-uh, you're not ready for that one yet (HG -- Fingers)." Or this part of me doesn't want to know about that yet. *(This theme of parts missing is Mineral Kingdom, as he is not in battle to survive which would be Animal Kingdom. This theme of missing parts and identity is the 3rd row periodic table.)*

The reason I went like this *(HG)* is because it's in me. I feel like it's all inside me. It's in here *(HG to head)*, or wherever. I'm not seeing it as an external thing so much. It's an internal sense, like a hazy area of myself. It's like there's a part of me that I can't connect to. *(He differentiates that it is not Animal Kingdom (victim/aggressor) but rather Mineral Kingdom (about parts of his existence). He has all the parts – just can't connect to some of them.)*

I've put a lot of trust in my mental capacities. I see that my mental has got me through life—that's my inner belief. *(Indicates that he is not lacking, so we are hearing center to right side of periodic table.)*

Being able to talk well, being able to understand things quickly, being able to communicate, having quite a vivid imagination. As an architect, it helps. (*For him, mental capacity is about his identity, about being able to talk, understand, communicate. This is Row 3.)*

I think for me the ego is kind of my sense of self that I've created over the years. You know, the architect, the Englishman, the whatever. I don't know. Whatever my picture of myself is, this is for me the ego. *(Row 3 is about ego development and identification, center to right side of periodic table.*)

I would like not to have these mental labels, just to explore, because the label can be just as much an imprisonment as it can be a help. (*Chlorum theme: don't put me in a box.*)
It's an easy example for me, that if I tell you I'm an architect, then you think of me as an architect. Whereas for me, inside myself, this is where I keep trying to get back to what makes me like I am. I am interested in getting closer to the real me, and when I say the real me, I mean not just this mental construct of "this is who I am". (*Scholten's delusional picture of Chlorum.*)

Source Language:

It's fuzzy, it's not clear. It's…this is (*HG Fingers*) fuzziness.
It's like hazy, it's like wanting, foggy, misty, opaque.
I think the actual definition of the pressing a panic button or clicking the light-switch, if I feel into the action more concretely, is actually like a fog rising up around me… It's dense, it has a heaviness. Thick, clammy.
Yes, and then I have this image, as the fog is rising, it functions like a drug. I feel drugged when I get this tiredness. Like I feel drugged – whooff I'm gone. It really feels like I could have just had a shot in the arm, and then it's like…I'm gone. It is like if I imagine a tear gas or some kind of gas that creates an effect. It's like this fog rising has the effect of anesthesia, like I'm just out of the count completely.
It's like being injected with some kind of drug that puts me to sleep.

Energy Language:

And it presses the panic button, (*HG indicates*) which is what I referred to as the light-switch. And then suddenly, whoooooof, I'm falling asleep.

CASE 2

YOUNG WOMAN with MENSTRUAL CRAMPS	*ANALYSIS*
Homeopath: What brings you here today? What is bothering you?	
Client: Ever since the first time I got my period, when I was 13, I've had the vast majority of the time very bad cramps. That very first time my mother had to give me codeine --- she is a nurse --- to fall asleep. She experienced the exact same thing the entire time she had a period.	*Chief Complaint – Bad Cramps.*
Tell me more about this.	
The main experience, I have really bad pain, don't know how to describe it better, back pain as well. Very intense; not achy. I experience waves, *(hand gesture (HG))* strong month, weaker month, I do feel waves, ease up and can breathe a little easier. There have been sometimes I end up throwing up, just from the pain, I don't feel nauseated; gets so overwhelming and my body can't handle it anymore.	*FACT LEVEL* *Local Sensation and Hand Gesture*
I've done a lot trying to pay attention to the signals when my period is *(HG)* coming. It was hard; I was not very regular, I was given different prescriptions over the years. If you medicate too late, it doesn't have much of a chance to do anything, I was always trying to (*HG – hand like a ball*) feel the first pangs, so that I could take what I needed to take but at the time not wanting to be taking too much. That is where a lot of the anxiety comes, how do I manage this, going through so many prescriptions and manage it effectively?	*FACT LEVEL* *EMOTION LEVEL*
Right now, percocet was too strong; made me throw up. Half vicodin is working and it's helpful and it is	

YOUNG WOMAN with MENSTRUAL CRAMPS	*ANALYSIS*
nice; but on the other hand if I didn't have to take strong drugs, I'd appreciate that.	
How does it affect you – to have this really intense pain?	
There's definitely anxiety around it in terms of, when is it going to come. Partially because I am not regular; in general, I go more than 28 days, 30, 32. Last month, I went to 35 days. In the summer I was in a couple of weddings I was panicky, thinking "Am I going to get it at one of these weddings?" I would not able to go if it was bad. I don't go to work. I have to be in bed. Then I also kind of dreading that experience to go through it on a regular basis; It's very very painful. I haven't had to experience any other pain like that, when I am in the middle of it, I also feel frustrated (*HG*), hopeless (*HG*); not knowing how long I am going to have to deal with it. The current remedy isn't working; It's a frustration that I have to experience it.	*Fact and Emotional Level.*
Can you describe exactly how this feels for you, the pain?	
Pause.................. In terms of the intensity it comes in waves, if you think of the word cramp (*HG – like holding a ball)* there is that kind of (*HG*) sensation that feels like (*HG*) cramping waves, it comes up and breaks up; I don't know what is going in my body when that happens. I guess it feels sharp but it's not like shooting pain. More like a tight uncomfortable feeling. It is really painful. Some months, I have very little pain. This discomfort type (same cramp HG) cramp, is not as painful, but it feels really annoying, so --- not like me --- so bothersome. Not really PMS. I experience being more emotional a week before and during the first day. The cramps themselves last the first 24, maybe 36 hours. Not all of that as intense. Usually is a	*Local Sensation* *Fact Level*

YOUNG WOMAN with MENSTRUAL CRAMPS	*ANALYSIS*
matter of getting through the first 12 hours or 8 hours. After that, I had to maintain a lower dose and if I didn't I may regret it. I was kind of in the clear to a certain extend. There have been times it started not as intense and gotten worse. Used to always start at certain times of day... Now I can't remember. I think it used to always start at either first thing in the morning, now it starts in the afternoon, then it is OK. Now, that shifted some, too. Those kinds of things are frustrating. I'm trying to understand it and be able to manage it accurately, and not having to have the experience of going to work and not be able to drive home. But also not staying at home when I feel fine instead of having to take the day off.	
Describe this cramping and gesture (HG) that is repeated a lot, waves, breaks...?	
When I'm talking about it being in waves, at the down times sometimes I associate it (*HG*) with everything being tight in my stomach and then it releases and everything stops. And that's when the pain goes away some.	
Describe this cramping and this release gesture (HG)?	
Another piece that's important for you to understand: when I have really bad pain, a sound, a touch even lovingly, is painful. I always experience it as everything that makes my (*HG*) muscles tense; really hurts (*HG – repeated HG*). I can't relax them. My mom advises me to relax; when the body is tensing up (*same HG*) you can't get rid of pain. She tries to get me to lie flat; could imagine it would help the process, using the heating pad, keep my muscles relaxed. How long could I stay like that? I end up tightening up; I get frustrated, making it worse, once I end up tightening up I start moving around, I could never stop. None of it is helping	*This repeated Gesture with Energy is the Vital Expression.* *This is a common symptom of cramps but since it keeps coming together, we follow:* *Tensing/ tight cramp vs. Release/ relax* *We will follow even though common, because they have energy for her.* *Moving around comes in as an aspect of the Vital Expression along with Tightening, Tense, Cramp, Release and Relax.*

YOUNG WOMAN with MENSTRUAL CRAMPS	*ANALYSIS*
me feel better; feels like all my muscles tense up and I can't...	
Tensing, tight, cramp. Release, relax?	
I was on an airplane; I did have the medication but not my heating pad, I always use a heating pad. The pain was getting really bad, I was pretty panicked. Talked to flight attendant to help me. I just told myself, "This month, mind over matter." I sat still. I remember holding on the bottle of medicine, trying to stay still, deal with it mentally as best as I could. That month I did make it, the pain didn't get worse. It worked then. I use my mind separately, how I separate mentally and emotionally.	*Miasm Hint* *Now "Stay still" comes in....*
What does this mean?	
That means, the entire time I am experiencing the pain I am thinking about what I could have done to avoid it. Sometimes for instance, I end up throwing up, at times when I feel like (*HG*), the pain is really bad, there is no way to get out of it, oh my God it hurts so much (*HG*). I almost feel certain to a certain extent I play a role, to the point where I get myself to throw up. So I'm saying to myself "no you aren't going through a violent experience with the body;" doesn't help the cramps at all, so I obviously don't if I don't have to. It freaks me out.	*All about the PAIN...*
How does it freak you out?	
I always hated throwing up since I was little, pretty unpleasant. There was something scary about being out of control of your body, and then physically the sensation is unpleasant, the way your body is convulsing and then the taste in your mouth. To a certain extent, it's layering on top of the worse thing I'm experiencing something else I can't stand experiencing. I feel physically worse. I threw up	*Dropped into Emotion Level.* *Miasm Hint* *Story.......*

YOUNG WOMAN with MENSTRUAL CRAMPS	*ANALYSIS*
too, first month at college. Ended up throwing up in the trash. The first month was the hardest, I didn't have my mom, it was definitely a very painful month. And to be throwing up in trash can in the dorm room, I was definitely feeling a lot of self pity that month.	
I want to take you back to this cramping, tightness and then the release that happens sometimes. You did this (*HG*). Just more words for that.	*Go back to the Vital Expression...*
It feels like <u>tightening</u> but it's also all over. It definitely feels like it's <u>all over my body,</u> but this whole area is affected, it's not like it's localized in a particular spot. I do feel it in my back, but it's not a typical back ache, much more intense than that.	*Local Sensation.* *Cramp, Tightening...*
More words – define?	
It's as if <u>all of my insides are pulling and pushing and moving around</u>, my muscles are kind of <u>overly sensitive,</u> the muscles in stomach and back, are (*HG*) all like <u>contracting, or contracted and I can't let them release</u>. I mean it doesn't feel the same as if right now I could contract my stomach muscles, it doesn't feel like that... It's just as...	*Kingdom Language:* *Tight, Cramp, Still, Pull, Push, Contracting, Tense, Holding.* *Relax, Release, Breaks, Moving Around.* *Repeated Sensation and it's Opposite – always telling us the same thing.* *Confirmation is this huge consuming issue with Pain and Sensitivity =* *PLANT KINGDOM.*
It's as if?	*Vital Expression in Plants is often the Sensation of the Plant Family.* *Similar to Cactus –Anacardiae but the opposites don't fit?.............*

YOUNG WOMAN with MENSTRUAL CRAMPS	*ANALYSIS*
It's as if when you picture doctors pour a liquid to see inside and it becomes a different color. It's as if they pour that through this whole section, whatever. It causes you pain, seeping through all of this area, doing damage somehow...	*Confirmed Kingdom – Let's go to Source.*
Describe that image as much as you can?	*Damage common to plants.*
I guess if I think of that, then it's a matter of either trying to figure out if I'm going to wait until it drains out of me. Sloshes inside of me, overpowers me. At times I feel there's nothing I can do; it is inside me. No way to get it out.	*Since we know the kingdom, we can ignore this or just pursue it to confirm...*
How do you experience this liquid, that's causing the damage and causing the pain?	
I experience it as doing physical damage to me, not severe damage. But damage as in general quality of life. I have to worry about what impact it will have on me each time it is inside of me, or each time I experience that.	*Damage is Plant.......* *Inside Me – hints Plant as well.*
And the sensation of this inside of you is what?	
Pain, I feel like the whole thing. There aren't enough words for pain. Pain. I either wait for it to go away or try to strategize and make it go away. No way to have an impact on what is happening.	
Contracting and Tighening or Release, and it Breaks. Describe a little bit more what happens and the opposite of the cramping.	
Sometimes the release is very short; and it almost immediately goes into the cramping. It does feel like some kind of (HG) tightening. There is this tight... ball. There is this tightening and then it explodes, not in a dramatic way, and it releases. It will either be a momentary release or it will release	*Seeping, Drains out, Slosh out, Pulling, Tightening, Explodes, Release*

YOUNG WOMAN with MENSTRUAL CRAMPS	*ANALYSIS*
for two minutes or half hour. In those moments, I'm amazed of feeling normal. Feeling my stomach is my own again, I can breathe again, things are not reacting to every turn and touch in the same way, there is what I take for granted when I feel fine. When it is in comparison to how it's been it feels like a release (*HG*). I feel maybe there is almost a sensation of warmth.	*Warmth*
Describe Relaxed State.	**As we continue through the case, asking about generals, dreams, fears, etc., nothing else emerges, just a lot of story.** **We ask about everything, and there are not enough SRP's to repertorize to get the remedy.** **We NEED the SOURCE.** **We patiently listen and ask until we get to a place of source language.**
The stomach is relaxed; in the relaxed state I feel like my stomach is calm, this whole region. There are times that it isn't as distinct as contract and release. There are times when I take medication, to be able to fall asleep. Those are the ideal times. The pain is bad, I take the medication and then I fall asleep. I wake up and the pain is under control. Weekends and evenings, I take the medication and go to bed. So there are times I don't feel the release, the experience. When the pain is over, emotionally there is kind of a release and relief, kind of connected in that way.	
Just use more words for that Release?	
Relaxing of the muscles. I was at work, I was definitely going through the waves quite a bit, experiencing the waves. Nerve racking. The next wave would be much worse. I was trying to figure out: "Do I need to go home, or go to my volunteer thing?" There was a moment when the pain was gone and I was just sitting there trying to figure out how I felt...	

YOUNG WOMAN with MENSTRUAL CRAMPS	*ANALYSIS*
The moment the pain was gone, how did it feel?	
It is like the calm returned. My stomach and the rest of my body is calm. It is that kind of, there is so much relief I feel normal. Feels better than normal. Feels good. "Oh, I have my body back." It is definitely interesting. I always experience the waves like this *(HG)* or like this *(HG)*. When they let up I can breathe, relax. To a certain extent, the pain is really bad. It is so much work to manage it. I don't know what I can do. When the pain initially starts it usually comes in twinges. Sometimes I feel the pain the day before I get the period or really get the cramps. I used to always get it in the morning, when I woke up, in the shower I'd think it is coming, these twinges, tightening up in my stomach. Is it really happening? It will come the next morning, and so the twinges start until it gets to the real peak and the pain is longer. Sometimes it's pretty quick, not much time to react, before the pain. When I experience the pain, I feel like my senses are very sensitive, senses are sensitive basically to noise, touch, definitely because when any of my muscles contract it makes the pain that much worse, throughout the experience of the pain it is always in waves. I would say some months, I get some kind of break from the pain until the medication times out. Other months, there are more waves, more back and forth experiences and tightening and releasing some, and then typically ends if the medication has worked or if enough time has passed. Usually the medication ends up being a piece of it. Doesn't help in the worst part of pain. Helps with the lesser pains. If it's the right kind of medication, it helps to cut if off earlier and not experience it as much.	
A little bit about this sensitivity to sound and touch. How do you experience it?	
It's very frustrating. You can't make the world stop	

YOUNG WOMAN with MENSTRUAL CRAMPS	*ANALYSIS*
just because you have your cramps. That's another frustrating piece of it. I used to experience it more intensely; in the grand scheme, the pain and the cramps have decreased some since my teenage and college years. That used to be another whole reason I wouldn't want to be out and about, driving would be awful; the break noises, it was just you don't realize you <u>react</u> to the noise (*HG*). Painful; some would be painful. My mom, or whoever, I'd be like "Please don't sit on the side of bed, 'cause the bed is going to shift. And then I'm going to tense up and it is going to kill. Talk to me quietly." She got to the point where she would know, <u>test the water</u>, talk quietly, see if I needed help, to see if I needed a heating pad, tea. If I couldn't respond to her she'd know. It was <u>too painful talking to me, too painful</u> to talk in response. She would come back later... Yea...	
What dreams do you get?	
I don't remember a lot of dreams in general. I don't really have... My dreams always tend to be (*HG*) kind of nonsensical, there's a person from this environment and that environment and that happens for a little bit of time. Not narratives. Just kind of bunch of weird stuff: kindergarden teacher and a frog... One time I can really think of, I went through a very difficult break up with my girlfriend for five years, clear narrative this was happening. This was the conversation, this outcome, for an extended period of time, many nights, after we first broke up... What was the feeling? It was <u>painful draining</u>. It felt frustrating, what was already so difficult during my awake hours was following me in my sleeping hours. My troubles now following me that I remember when I wake up, I think, "Did I have dreams?" Remembering emotional things throws you off; when you wake up, it feels like it happened. Any experience you had, you had to deal with the emotion of it (*HG*). Get back to where you are in your awake life. Painful. Let me give a brief story. My girlfriend and I had been together	

YOUNG WOMAN with MENSTRUAL CRAMPS	*ANALYSIS*
for four-and-a-half years. Moved out to Minnesota after four years. After six months, for a complicated set of reasons she broke up with me, didn't have to do with our relationship. *(HG)* Job stuff. I all of a sudden, felt I had to move back to Boston, did not have enough of a support structure set up for me out there to go through something like this. I had to leave a job I loved, left the apartment, moved back. I didn't have the relationship or job any more, or any one to talk to seriously about having a huge family loss. It was really difficult, painful, sad. I still have a lot of sadness, pain, still pretty sad.	*ALL ABOUT PAIN!!!*
Describe this pain, how do you experience this kind of pain?	
It is hard. Incredulous that everything happened, and that she was able to throw out every thing we had built up and moving towards. It is hard. We are now back in touch. I came back, and it will be two years. The first year, didn't have any contact. Since last fall, we've been in contact. It has been really good. Whereas before there was no contact, it felt almost like a death; lose the person completely. There is the possibility of having her in my life but the difficulty of that is that is not in a way I had wanted for so long, like us to be in a realitonship that we are not. If I was in another relationship, look back wanting that one. In that case was good, and miss that legitimately strong connection. I think there is a piece of it that feels kind of tragic in the sense of the relationship was so good. Made us both happy, had our families involved, plans for the future couldn't work out, things outside of *(HG)* the relationship couldn't get along.	
So what are these things outside of the relationship? What is this (HG)?	
Things. The issues she had to deal with and the	

YOUNG WOMAN with MENSTRUAL CRAMPS	*ANALYSIS*
reason why she broke up with me were coming out to her parents; her relationship with her parents; had not grown in the way she wanted to; still felt close if she could fully let herself be honest with them. Also (*HG*) issues of her adoption, still had no contact with birth parents. Having no information about her birth parents was having an impact on her happiness, her ability to be in a relationship. Some of it was work related, work-life balance, she is a basketball coach on Division 1, crazy hours, very demanding, her wanting to know she had not sacrificed for something she might have been able to do in the future like a career etc. It didn't feel fair. Just hard to understand why it had to happen. We were both happy together, in love. Wanted the samc thing for the future. I know I had a very blessed and priveleged life. Nobody wants to deal with why did I deserve this big piece (HG), the control piece, it is always uncomforable. I <u>don't feel I have the ability to be in control in my life, my body</u>, maybe in the case of my girlfriend, it is much more. Doesn't matter that I love her. This is another individual. I don't have the control to change it, I have to let go of that, (*HG*). That's been a lot of what the learning has been for me. I think I have grown some, around that whole issue, I have a little more peace, going through the loss, not being in touch, not getting the response, deal again with not having to keep control of the situation. In terms of the cramps, the physical pain is obviously terrible but the fact that <u>I can't manage it, I can't contol it, I can't be in control</u>, can't help myself, it's a big piece of the emotionally negative part for me.	*Cancer Miasm* *Miasm off the CC*
What kind of fears do you have? Or even as a child what fears did you have?	
I don't have any. I don't have any of those fears like being afraid of bridges. Don't have any of those. The fears that affect me most are fears of losing people I love, I'd say that's probably the number one.	

YOUNG WOMAN with MENSTRUAL CRAMPS	*ANALYSIS*
As a kid?	
I can remember as a kid the nights my mom worked late I couldn't fall asleep (*HG*) until she came home. My mind would race. If she came home a little later than she was supposed to, what could have happenend, maybe she won't come home, that kind of thing. I am an only child. I am sure all kids potentially imagined that experience. Very close to both my parents, very central to my life.	
I'm just going to take you back to just (*HG*) throwing up. When things go out then the throwing up is even worse. Just describe one more time in the worst case scenario when you do throw up...	*Had a lot of energy...*
The months when the pain is really bad, there were times when I've ended throwing up. It doesn't start from a separate feeling of nausea, it starts from the pain and the pain ends up making me feel nauseous (*HG*). I almost feel sick. There is something <u>rising</u> up, almost the sensation of something rising before I will be able to keep that down or not. At times I am able to calm myself and not throw up, usually by taking my mind someplace else, like "don't think about it and maybe you're not going to throw up" versus the times when I'm going "Oh my God I am going to throw up" *(HG)* and it just feels like the fact that I'm going to throw up it kind of rises in me before the actual throw up <u>rises in me</u>.	
This rising, just give more words, for the rising that happens?	
It is kind of like to a certain extent a sensation or idea that I am going to throw up (*HG*). The thought, <u>grows</u> and becomes a reality, whatever first strikes me, "Oh my God is so bad I feel sick and it caught me." It is going to happen. It has caught me, kind of beyond the point I can go back.	

YOUNG WOMAN with MENSTRUAL CRAMPS	*ANALYSIS*
And the opposite of that?	
Letting down, relaxing, exhaling, tightening up, inhaling nervousness, just discomfort anxiety.	*ALL CONFIRMS BACK*
Not so much in your life but in general what comes to mind, letting down, relaxing, exhaling, tightening up, inhaling, nervousness, anxiety? Any color, any shape? What is going on in the imagination?	*Case starts coming back here...*
My favorite color for the release, calm, comfort, is BLUE. The first thing I thought of was red which is appropriate given the blood, it reminds me of things I don't think regularly at different times, the difficulty around my period. I think what that means for the future, trouble having kids, and have that worry on a regular basis. My mom had two miscarriages. She had me at 41. She had one before and one afterwards.	
(*HG*) – JUST THIS and THIS? Whatever comes to mind with these two?	
This tightening inhaling discomfort would connect more broadly in terms of my emotions over my life, it would connect more times when I am not as at ease, at times when I worry and I am uncomfortable with people I am around, worried nervous, and don't feel safe. As opposed to when I do feel safe, at ease and supported, I can just relax and be completely myself, physically comfortable (HG) in my environment, my body is strong, part of who I am, an asset, not causing me a problem.	
In your imagination – something in the world that has this quality?	*Desperate Question??? Must LISTEN for WHAT DOESN'T FIT!! Not Easy for Her..........*

YOUNG WOMAN with MENSTRUAL CRAMPS	*ANALYSIS*
	Let her PAUSE....................
Someting just popped into my head --------- but it's not quite right. Something just came to me like the sea or the ocean, but I'm not quite sure if this is what I was thinking about, they are seaweed pictures -- and then I'm back to the wave thing -- of water moves in and out, there is some kind of plant closes up and opens up, but the wave comes in and releases as the water goes out (*HG*). Do you know what I'm talking about?	*All the Words and Ideas Come in Here:* *Waves, Closes Up, Releases. Closes In..........* *LIST OUT THESE WORDS*
Waves, closes up, releases, closes in... Can you describe it a little bit more?	
Definitely sea weed, long strings, leaves that kind of come together and form a flowering type shape but then open out and flatten, water goes out, waves, closes and it opens up, color dark green, bright pink.	
In your imagination – how do you experience the water coming in and going out?	
First thing it doesn't make sense. It feesl like supported and closed up. It would feel good and safe and then water feels, ugh, falling out. Nothing supporting; kind of opposite of what I was describing. Not my first though. It could be when water it is too much. It is crushing, not really getting crushed, (*HG*) goes out, the water is able to release, not pushed around. **We stopped the case here and had her draw it -- -- interesting, the waves.**	*Water Falling Out (Drain), Release, Push.....* *SHE DRAWS IT – IT COMES TOGETHER and FLOWS OUT.*
Is there any thing else?	

YOUNG WOMAN with MENSTRUAL CRAMPS	*ANALYSIS*
There are a few random things. The back pain I mentioned to you. I hold stress in my back and stress at different points, knots and tension, (*HG*). My mom has always had back and neck problems. Our bodies are very similar. We have the same frame too, I am a little like her, and she has the nerve sciatica. There have been times I've had long drives with a clutch and I've had my left leg out for three hours straight. Seems to me my sciatica nerve gets bothered by that, lower back pain, pain wrapping around my hip, and goes down my left leg, really bad. Different back issues at different points. I also clench and grind my teeth at night; I have some TMJ stuff going on at night. I get some popping in and out. Depends how stressed I am; I literally can't get past this. I have to hold my mouth if it starts aching. On the left side more. That whole thing stresses me out, doing damage. There is a tooth up here that my dentist told me recently is probably cracked from the grinding. Nothing I can do about it. I am asleep, so what am I suppose to do? Retainers and mouth guards stand it in place. My mom grinds her teeth. Mouth guard is so annoying and uncomfortable. The retainer is better than that. I did have cysts on my breast, sensitivity. I had pain particularly around my period, with swelling in my breast. All tiny, pea-sized. Nothing could be done. I check them; they may go away. The pain has decreased from that; it was annoying. The only other thing that is bothering me is that maybe I am getting a bunion, on my left foot. And the cysts, the pain was mostly on the left, in the breast. I wear high heels at work. It really depends on what kind of shoes I'm wearing (*HG*). It is very sensitive when I take off my shoes. Even when I start walking the bending at that joint is painful. I am getting worried about it. A friend had surgery; 8 weeks recovery. I am 27; she is 65. In general, my experience is that I am very healthy. I grew up as an athlete, love being active and I think I have a very positive relationship with my body. I see it as a source of strength. I feel very blessed with no health problems.	*Can't control.*

YOUNG WOMAN with MENSTRUAL CRAMPS	*ANALYSIS*
Foods?	
I definitely have a sweet tooth. Am a carb person. I don't worry about my weight. I am aware, needing to think long term cardiovascular, sodium longer term. I love eating bread, pasta, cereal, those are the tings I really enjoy, actually fill me up, I don't always eat, pretty fast metabolism, I can eat consistently.	
Dislike?	
There's a lot of vegetables I don't really like. I don't like fish, I like sea food but no fish, some vegetables I like.	
Do you tend to be thirsty?	
Not so thirsty. I need to drink at same time I eat, always thirsty when eating. Just drinking water? Why would I want to do it? It has no taste. I force myself to drink it, except when I exercise.	
Do you tend to be more warm or cold?	
C: Cold, cold, cold. I love the summer when it's not cold.	
Do you perspire a lot or not so much?	
Not so much. Mainly when I am stressed, like I am about to do a presentation, something out of the ordinary. Otherwise, when I'm exercising. Probably on the normal or lower I guess. I have scoliosis. They found it later on, there's nothing I need to do. I do sit ups. You can see it. I never noticed if it had some impact on my back, I was never able to associate it, if I had any back pain that it had	

YOUNG WOMAN with MENSTRUAL CRAMPS	*ANALYSIS*
anything to do with that.	
	Remedy: fucus vesiculosus (sea weed) Potency: 200C

ADDITIONAL NOTES:

Client: young woman with severe menstrual cramps

Overview: Client describes menstrual cramps with common language (tense, tight, cramp, release, relax) but with a lot of energy and a much-repeated gesture. Repeated sensation and its opposite, always telling us the same thing: this huge consuming issue with pain and sensitivity. This indicates Plant Kingdom. Subkingdom was not clear, with few rubrics to work with, so had to really push client to source to identify. There are not many sea weed remedies.

Chief Complaint: menstrual cramps

Vital Expression: HG (like holding a ball), cramps, tense, tight

Some questions homeopath asks:

How does it affect you to have this really intense pain?

Can you describe what this pain is for you – use as many words as possible.

Describe this cramping and HG that is repeated a lot, waves, break . . .

You are doing great, this is what I need. So there is this tight, cramping and if you start moving around it breaks, releases and then if you could really relax the pain would. .?

It's as if . . ?

How do you experience this liquid, seeping, causing damage and pain?

In your imagination – is there something in the world that has this quality of cramping and release you could give as an example? (desperate question)

Kingdom Language: Plant Kingdom
It is all my inside pulling and pushing and moving around, my muscles are kind of overly sensitive the muscles in stomach and back, are **HG** all like contracting, contracted let them release, if I am ok not contract my stomach muscles.
. . .when doctors pour liquid to see inside different color pour that through whole section whatever pour into you cause you pain seeping in all this area, doing damage.
The release is very short, immediately goes into the cramping, there is this tight ball . . . it explodes not in a dramatic way, more of a release.

Source Language:
Popped into my head - it is not quite right something like the sea or ocean what I was thinking of it, they are seaweed pictures -- back to the wave thing - definitly sea weed long strings leaves whatever kind of coming flowering type shape but then open out and flatten water goes out, waves closes and it opens up. Color dark green, bright pink

Energy Language:
Water moves in and out, there is some kind of plant closes up and opens up, the waves comes in and releases out HG

Miasm: Cancer
There was something scary about being out of control of your body.
The control piece, it is always uncomfortable I don't feel I have the ability to be in control in my life, my body.

Remedy: fucus vesiculosus (seaweed)

Dose: 200C

K. HOMEWORK

Please submit three paper cases. Circle or highlight all the kingdom language and identify, which kingdom you think it is, as well as the level you think the patient is expressing the ideas.

For feedback you can send or email your homework to:

Melissa Burch, CCH
Inner Health, Inc.
175 Harvey Street, Unit 13
Cambridge, MA 02140 USA

617-491-3374

melissa@innerhealth.us

About Melissa Burch, CCH

Melissa Burch, CCH, co-founded The Catalyst School of Homeopathy with Christopher Beaver, CCH. She established live phone case supervision and clinics based on the Sensation Method.

She created a unique homeopathic phone referral service with a homeopath team approach. She is president of Inner Health, Inc., which produces numerous online and onsite courses for homeopaths, homeopathic patients and people interested in alternative medicine. She produced the first Radio Series on Homeopathy.

She was the Master Homeopath for the proving of Stoichactis Kenti Sea Anemone. She co-wrote and published the five part "Vital Sensation Manual." Ms. Burch worked with Dr. Nandita Shah at Quiet Healing Center in South India for over a year and half. She graduated from the School of Homeopathy New York, directed by Jo Daly, and the New York School of Homeopathy, directed by Robert Stewart.

About Inner Health, Inc.

Inner Health (IH) provides homeopathic services to the general public and to the homeopathic community. IH is a leader in establishing the highest quality of services in the complementary and alternative medical field through its education, practitioners, workshops and services.

IH's vision is to make homeopathy a household word. Our goal is to identify IH in the consumer's mind as the place to go for the best, natural deep healing on all level—mental, emotional, physical and spiritual; and to create a demand for homeopathy and in particular for Certified IH Homeopaths, through our innovative, educational and creative marketing materials.

Training

IH provides basic and post-graduate training for homeopaths to develop reliable and better results in their practices by following the IH Approach—a systematic way of case taking and analysis based on the Sensation Method—and by implementing the IH System, which includes case management protocols, scripts and information, client business services and marketing.

Homeopaths have the opportunity to train and become Certified IH Homeopaths through workshops, supervision and educational materials. Combined with our own extensive marketing of IH and the IH approach to homeopathy, which results in constant referrals to Certified IH Homeopaths, IH Homeopaths will have a unique and wonderful opportunity to develop themselves as professional homeopaths, heal others, share clinical information with the homeopathic community, be well paid and have excellent systems to guide them to provide the highest care to the client.